Copyright ©

Contents

Introduction

The Volumetrics Diet is a unique approach to weight loss that focuses on consuming low-calorie, high-volume foods. Developed by Barbara Rolls, a nutrition researcher and professor at Penn State University, this diet plan promotes the idea that people can eat more and feel satisfied while still losing weight.

Highlight its effectiveness in weight loss

The effectiveness of the Volumetrics Diet lies in its emphasis on consuming foods that are low in energy density. Energy density refers to the number of calories contained in a specific amount of food. High-energy-density foods, such as those that are rich in fats and sugars, tend to have a high number of calories per gram, which can contribute to weight gain. On the other hand, low-energy-density foods have a lower number of calories per gram, allowing you to eat a larger portion while still consuming fewer calories.

By incorporating low-energy-density foods into your meals, the Volumetrics Diet helps you feel fuller and satisfied without overeating. These foods typically have a high water content, such as fruits and vegetables, which adds bulk to your meals without significantly increasing the calorie content. As a result, you can eat a greater volume of food while keeping your calorie intake in check, leading to weight loss.

Mention the focus on consuming low-calorie, high-volume foods

The core principle of the Volumetrics Diet revolves around choosing foods that are low in calorie density but high in volume. This means opting for nutrient-rich foods that provide a satisfying eating experience while keeping the calorie count low.

Fruits and vegetables are the stars of the Volumetrics Diet. They are naturally low in calories and high in water content, which means you can enjoy larger portions without consuming excessive calories. These colorful and flavorful plant-based foods not only provide essential vitamins, minerals, and antioxidants but also contribute to feelings of fullness and satiety.

In addition to fruits and vegetables, the Volumetrics Diet encourages the consumption of other low-calorie, high-volume foods. This includes lean proteins such as poultry, fish, and legumes, which are filling and provide essential nutrients without adding excess calories. Whole grains like brown rice, quinoa, and whole wheat bread are also recommended due to their fiber content and ability to keep you satisfied for longer periods.

The Volumetrics Diet also encourages reducing the consumption of high-energy-density foods, such as those that are high in added sugars, unhealthy fats, and refined grains. These foods tend to be calorie-dense and can lead to weight gain when consumed in large amounts. By limiting their intake, you create space in your diet for healthier, low-calorie options.

In conclusion, the Volumetrics Diet offers an effective approach to weight loss by focusing on consuming low-calorie, high-volume foods. By incorporating water-rich fruits and vegetables, lean proteins, whole grains, and other nutrient-dense foods, you can create a satisfying and balanced eating plan that promotes weight loss without the need for strict calorie counting or deprivation. Remember, it's not just about the quantity of food you eat, but also the quality.

Understanding the Volumetrics Approach

A. Explain the energy density concept (calories per gram of food)

The Volumetrics Diet is built upon the concept of energy density, which refers to the number of calories contained in a specific weight or volume of food. Energy density is measured in calories per gram (or calories per 100 grams) of food. Understanding energy density is crucial because it helps individuals make informed choices about the foods they consume in order to achieve weight loss.

B. Differentiate between low-energy-density and high-energy-density foods

Low-energy-density foods are those that contain relatively fewer calories per gram. These foods tend to be high in water content and/or fiber, which adds volume without significantly increasing the calorie count. Examples of low-energy-density foods include most fruits and vegetables, broth-based soups, and non-starchy vegetables like leafy greens. These foods provide a sense of fullness and satisfaction while allowing for a larger portion size due to their lower calorie content.

On the other hand, high-energy-density foods are those that contain more calories per gram. These foods are often rich in fats, sugars, or refined carbohydrates, which contribute to their higher caloric value. Examples of high-energy-density foods include fried snacks, sweets, pastries, fatty meats, and full-fat dairy products. These foods tend to be more calorie-dense and can quickly add up in terms of calorie intake without providing the same level of satiety.

C. Discuss the satiety factor and how it contributes to weight loss

Satiety refers to the feeling of fullness and satisfaction after a meal. It plays a crucial role in weight management because it helps control hunger and prevents overeating. The Volumetrics Diet capitalizes on the satiety factor by encouraging the consumption of low-energy-density foods that provide a greater volume of food for fewer calories.

Low-energy-density foods, such as fruits, vegetables, and foods high in fiber, are not only nutrient-rich but also take up more space in the stomach. When you consume these foods, they stretch the stomach receptors, triggering signals to the brain that you are full and satisfied. This helps prevent overeating and reduces the likelihood of consuming excess calories.

In contrast, high-energy-density foods tend to be less filling and can leave you wanting more. These foods often lack the volume and fiber content found in low-energy-density options, leading to a quicker consumption and potential overeating.

By incorporating low-energy-density foods into your meals, the Volumetrics Diet enhances satiety, allowing you to feel satisfied while consuming fewer calories. This approach helps create a calorie deficit, which is essential for weight loss. Additionally, the emphasis on consuming nutrient-rich foods ensures that you receive essential vitamins, minerals, and other beneficial compounds while working towards your weight loss goals.

Understanding the energy density concept and the role of satiety in the Volumetrics Diet enables individuals to make informed choices when selecting their meals and snacks. By prioritizing low-energy-density foods that provide a greater volume and a sense of fullness, you can create a sustainable and effective approach to weight

loss without feeling deprived or hungry.

Volumetrics Diet Review: Does It Work for Weight Loss?

The Volumetrics Diet is an eating plan designed to promote weight loss by having you fill up on low calorie, nutrient-dense foods.

It's meant to reduce feelings of hunger by prioritizing foods with a high water content and low calorie density. It also encourages other healthy habits, such as regular exercise and keeping a food journal.

Still, you may wonder whether it's a good fit for you.

This article provides a comprehensive review of the Volumetrics Diet, including its effectiveness for weight loss.

DIET REVIEW SCORECARD

- Overall score: 3.0

- Weight loss: 2.5

- Healthy eating: 3.5

- Sustainability: 3.5

- Whole body health: 3.5

- Nutrition quality: 2.0

- Evidence-based: 3.0

BOTTOM LINE: The Volumetrics Diet emphasizes foods with a low calorie density, which can increase weight loss and improve overall diet quality. However, it restricts some healthy food groups and is time-intensive.

Share on Pinterest

What is the Volumetrics Diet?

The Volumetrics Diet claims to help you feel full while eating fewer calories.

It's based on a book by nutrition scientist Dr. Barbara Rolls, which provides in-depth guidelines, recipes, and information on how to calculate the calorie density of your favorite foods.

The diet encourages you to eat nutrient-dense foods that are low in calories and high in water, such as fruits, vegetables, and soups. Meanwhile, it limits calorie-dense foods like cookies, candies, nuts, seeds, and oils.

Dr. Rolls asserts that these restrictions help you feel fuller for longer, cut your calorie intake, and promote weight loss.

Unlike other diets, the Volumetrics Diet is intended to foster healthy eating habits and should be viewed as a long-term lifestyle change rather than a short-term solution.

SUMMARY

The Volumetrics Diet prioritizes low calorie, nutrient-dense foods with a high water content, which is thought to help keep you feeling full to encourage weight loss.

How it works

The Volumetrics Diet groups foods into four categories based on their calorie density:

- Category 1 (very low calorie density): calorie density of less than 0.6

- Category 2 (low calorie density): calorie density of 0.6–1.5

- Category 3 (medium calorie density): calorie density of 1.6–3.9

- Category 4 (high calorie density): calorie density of 4.0–9.0

Dr. Rolls's book provides detailed information on how to calculate calorie density. In general, you should divide the number of calories in a particular serving size by its weight in grams. You'll end up with a figure between 0 and 9.

Foods with a high water content, such as broccoli, typically score very low in calorie density, while desserts and processed foods like dark chocolate usually rank high.

A typical meal on the Volumetrics Diet should mostly comprise foods from Category 1, as well as include foods from Category 2 to help round out your plate. You can eat small amounts of foods from Category 3 and very limited portions from Category 4.

The diet's standard meal plan provides around 1,400 calories per day but can be adjusted to fit your calorie goals by adding extra snacks or increasing portion sizes.

No foods are completely off-limits on the Volumetrics Diet. In fact, you can include foods with a high calorie density by modifying your portion sizes and adjusting your other meals.

Furthermore, the diet encourages at least 30–60 minutes of exercise each day.

You should keep track of your physical activity and food intake in a journal to monitor your progress and identify areas that may need improvement.

SUMMARY

The Volumetrics Diet categorizes foods based on their calorie density, prioritizing those that score very low. It also encourages you to get regular exercise, as well as log your food intake and physical activity.

Does it work for weight loss?

Although few studies have examined the Volumetrics Diet specifically, research suggests that its central tenets aid weight loss.

Promotes low calorie intake

Selecting foods with a low calorie density is particularly effective. Because these foods have a substantial volume but are low in calories, you can eat large servings without significantly increasing your calorie intake (1Trusted Source).

Notably, a review of 13 studies in 3,628 people tied foods with a lower calorie density to increased weight loss. Similarly, an 8-year study in over 50,000 women associated high-calorie-density foods with increased weight gain.

Choosing foods with a low calorie density may also help curb cravings and reduce appetite, which could boost weight loss.

A 12-week study in 96 women with excess weight and obesity found that meals with a lower calorie density led to decreased cravings, increased feelings of fullness, and reduced hunger.

In an older study in 39 women, participants ate 56% more calories when served a large portion of a high-calorie-density meal, compared with a smaller, low-calorie-density meal (5Trusted Source).

Encourages regular exercise

Exercise is another important component of the Volumetrics Diet.

The diet recommends getting at least 30–60 minutes of physical activity per day, which may increase weight loss and fat loss by raising your energy expenditure, or the number of calories burned during the day.

SUMMARY

The Volumetrics Diet encourages regular exercise and emphasizes foods with a low calorie density, which are effective strategies to increase weight loss and reduce hunger and cravings.

Other health benefits

The Volumetrics Diet may offer several other health benefits.

May boost diet quality

By encouraging healthy foods that are low in calories but high in fiber, vitamins, and minerals, the Volumetrics Diet may help increase your intake of key nutrients and protect against nutritional deficiencies.

What's more, some research links diets with a low calorie density to improved diet quality (8Trusted Source).

Limits processed foods

Although the Volumetrics Diet doesn't completely ban any foods, most processed foods have a high calorie density and should be restricted as part of the plan.

Processed foods are not only typically lacking in essential nutrients like fiber, protein, vitamins, and minerals but also usually higher in calories, fat, sugar, and sodium.

Furthermore, studies tie regular intake of processed foods to a higher risk of cancer, heart disease, and premature death).

Flexible and sustainable

Unlike most fad diets, the Volumetrics Diet should be viewed as a long-term lifestyle change.

It pushes you to become more aware of your eating habits and food choices, which can help you make healthier dietary decisions by prioritizing foods with a lower calorie density, such as fruits and vegetables.

Additionally, because no foods are banned on the diet, you can enjoy your favorite dishes by making modifications and adjustments to your diet.

This may make the Volumetrics Diet a good fit for people seeking some flexibility and a sustainable eating plan to follow long term.

SUMMARY

The Volumetrics Diet limits processed foods and may improve diet quality. It's also flexible and designed to be maintained long term.

Potential downsides

The Volumetrics Diet has a few drawbacks to be aware of.

Time-intensive with few online resources

The diet requires significant time and energy investments, which may make it untenable for some people.

In addition to finding recipes, planning meals, and calculating calorie density, you're supposed to prepare most of your meals and snacks at home. This may make the diet too restrictive for those with a busy lifestyle, cramped kitchen, or limited access to fresh produce.

Although some support groups and recipes are available, online apps and resources for the diet are somewhat limited.

In fact, you may need to purchase the book by Dr. Rolls to calculate your meals' calorie density and track your food intake effectively.

Limits healthy fats

The diet also restricts certain foods rich in healthy fats, including nuts, seeds, and oils.

These foods provide monounsaturated and polyunsaturated fats, which may reduce inflammation and safeguard against chronic conditions like heart disease (12Trusted Source, 13Trusted Source, 14Trusted Source).

Moreover, many nutritious eating patterns like the Mediterranean diet encourage you to eat these foods.

Places too much emphasis on calories

Given that the Volumetrics Diet is based on calorie density, high calorie foods are limited.

This means that nutritious, high calorie foods like avocados, nut butter, and whole eggs are limited, while processed, low calorie foods like fat-free salad dressing and diet ice cream are allowed due to their low calorie density.

Low calorie foods are often packed with added sugar and other unhealthy ingredients to enhance their taste. Just because something is low in calories doesn't mean it's healthy.

SUMMARY

The Volumetrics Diet is time-intensive, and online resources are somewhat limited. It also restricts foods high in healthy fats, including nuts, seeds, and oils.

Foods to eat and avoid

Rather than banning any foods entirely, the Volumetrics Diet divides them into four categories based on their calorie density.

Category 1

Foods in Category 1 have a very low calorie density and should comprise the majority of your diet. They include:

• Fruits: apples, oranges, pears, peaches, bananas, berries, and grapefruit

• Non-starchy vegetables: broccoli, cauliflower, carrots, tomatoes, zucchini, and kale

• Soups: broth-based soups like vegetable soup, chicken soup, minestrone, and lentil soup

• Nonfat dairy: skim milk and nonfat yogurt

- Beverages: water, black coffee, and unsweetened tea

Category 2

Foods in the second category have a low energy density and can be enjoyed in moderation. They include:

- Whole grains: quinoa, couscous, farro, buckwheat, barley, and brown rice

- Legumes: chickpeas, lentils, black beans, and kidney beans

- Starchy vegetables: potatoes, corn, peas, squash, and parsnips

• Lean proteins: skinless poultry, white fish, and lean cuts of beef or pork

Category 3

Foods in the third category are considered medium calorie density. While they're permitted, it's important to keep an eye on serving sizes. These foods include:

• Meat: fatty fish, poultry with the skin, and high fat cuts of pork and beef

• Refined carbs: white bread, white rice, crackers, and white pasta

• Full fat dairy: whole milk, full fat yogurt, ice cream, and cheese

Category 4

Foods in the final category are classified as high energy density. These foods contain lots of calories per serving and should be eaten sparingly. They include:

• Nuts: almonds, walnuts, macadamia nuts, pecans, and pistachios

• Seeds: chia seeds, sesame seeds, hemp seeds, and flax seeds

• Oils: butter, vegetable oil, olive oil, margarine, and lard

• Processed foods: cookies, candies, chips, pretzels, and fast food

SUMMARY

Foods with a very low calorie density include non-starchy veggies, broth-based soups, and fruits. These should comprise the bulk of your diet. Meanwhile, you should limit your intake of processed foods, nuts, seeds, and oils.

Sample 3-day meal plan

On the Volumetrics Diet, you should eat 3 meals per day, plus 2–3 snacks. Here's a 3-day sample menu:

Day 1

- Breakfast: oatmeal with fruit and a glass of skim milk

- Snack: carrots with hummus

- Lunch: grilled chicken with quinoa and asparagus

- Snack: sliced apples and light string cheese

- Dinner: baked cod with spiced vegetable couscous

Day 2

- Breakfast: nonfat yogurt with strawberries and blueberries

- Snack: a hard-boiled egg with tomato slices

- Lunch: turkey chili with kidney beans and vegetables

- Snack: a fruit salad with melon, kiwi, and strawberries

- Dinner: zucchini boats stuffed with ground beef, tomatoes, bell peppers, and marinara sauce

Day 3

- Breakfast: scrambled eggs with mushrooms, tomatoes, and onions, plus a slice of whole wheat toast

- Snack: a smoothie with skim milk, banana, and berries

- Lunch: chicken noodle soup with a side salad

- Snack: air-popped popcorn

- Dinner: whole grain pasta with turkey meatballs and sautéed vegetables

SUMMARY

The meal plan above provides some simple meal and snack ideas for the Volumetrics Diet.

The bottom line

The Volumetrics Diet prioritizes foods with a low calorie density and high volume. It promotes weight loss by enhancing feelings of fullness while reducing hunger and cravings.

It may also improve your diet quality by increasing your intake of nutrient-dense foods like fruits and vegetables.

However, the Volumetrics Diet also requires substantial time and energy, restricts several healthy foods, and offers limited online resources, which may make it unsuitable for some people.

13 Low-Calorie Foods That Are Surprisingly Filling

One of the most challenging aspects of weight loss is cutting back on calories.

Many low-calorie foods can leave you feeling hungry and unfulfilled between meals, making it much more tempting to overeat and indulge.

Fortunately, plenty of healthy foods exist that are both filling and low in calories.

Here are 13 low-calorie foods that are surprisingly filling.

1. Oats

Oats can be an excellent addition to a healthy weight loss diet.

They're not only low in calories but also high in protein and fiber that keep you feeling full.

A 1/2-cup (40-gram) serving of dry oats has just 148 calories but packs 5.5 grams of protein and 3.8 grams of fiber — both of which can have a significant impact on your hunger and appetite (1).

One study in 48 adults demonstrated that eating oatmeal increased feelings of fullness and reduced hunger and calorie intake at the next meal (2Trusted Source).

Another small study linked instant and old-fashioned oatmeal to significantly improved appetite control over a four-hour period compared to a ready-to-eat breakfast cereal (3Trusted Source).

SUMMARYOats, which are high in fiber and protein, work to reduce hunger, increase feelings of fullness and improve appetite control.

2. Greek Yogurt

Greek yogurt is a great source of protein that can help curb cravings and promote weight loss.

Though the exact numbers vary between brands and flavors, a 2/3-cup (150-gram) serving of Greek yogurt typically provides about 130 calories and 11 grams of protein (4).

One study in 20 women examined how a high-protein yogurt snack affected appetite compared to unhealthy high-fat snacks like chocolate or crackers.

Not only did women who ate yogurt experience less hunger, but they also consumed 100 fewer calories at dinner than those who ate crackers or chocolate (5Trusted Source).

Meanwhile, in another study in 15 women, high-protein Greek yogurt helped reduce hunger and increase feelings of fullness compared to lower-protein snacks (6Trusted Source).

SUMMARYGreek yogurt is high in protein and linked to less hunger, subdued calorie intake and increased feelings of fullness.

3. Soup

Though soup is often dismissed as little more than a light and simple side dish, it can be very satisfying.

In fact, some research suggests that soups may be more filling than solid foods — even if they have the same ingredients.

For example, one study in 12 people indicated that smooth soup slowed the emptying of the stomach and was more effective at promoting fullness than a solid meal or chunky soup (7Trusted Source).

In another study in 60 people, eating soup prior to a meal decreased total calorie intake at lunch by an impressive 20% (8Trusted Source).

Keep in mind that creamy soups and chowders — while filling — may also be high in calories.

Opt for a lighter broth- or stock-based soup to minimize calories and maximize fullness.

SUMMARYCertain types of soup can be low in calories and slow the emptying of your stomach while reducing total calorie intake.

4. Berries

Berries — including strawberries, blueberries, raspberries and blackberries — are loaded with vitamins, minerals and antioxidants that can optimize your health.

Their high fiber content also boosts weight loss and reduces hunger.

For example, 1 cup (148 grams) of blueberries supplies just 84 calories but packs 3.6 grams of fiber (9).

Berries are also a great source of pectin, a type of dietary fiber that has been shown to slow stomach emptying and increase feelings of fullness in human and animal studies (10Trusted Source, 11Trusted Source, 12Trusted Source).

This could also help cut calorie consumption to aid weight loss.

One study noted that a 65-calorie afternoon snack of berries decreased calorie intake later in the day compared to a 65-calorie confectionery snack (13Trusted Source).

SUMMARYBerries are high in fiber and pectin, which slow the emptying of your stomach and promote feelings of fullness.

5. Eggs

Eggs are extremely nutrient-dense, as they're low in calories but rich in many vital nutrients.

A single large egg has approximately 72 calories, 6 grams of protein and a wide array of important vitamins and minerals (14).

Studies suggest that starting your day with a serving of eggs can reduce hunger and boost fullness.

In a study in 30 women, those who ate eggs for breakfast instead of a bagel experienced greater feelings of fullness and consumed 105 fewer calories later in the day (15Trusted Source).

Other studies observe that a high-protein breakfast could decrease snacking, slow the emptying of your stomach and reduce levels of ghrelin, the hormone responsible for hunger (16Trusted Source, 17Trusted Source).

SUMMARYEggs are packed with protein and make a superb low-calorie breakfast choice.

6. Popcorn

Thanks to its high fiber content, popcorn tops the charts as one of the most filling low-calorie snacks.

Though there are only 31 calories in 1 cup (8 grams) of air-popped popcorn, it boasts

1.2 grams of dietary fiber — up to 5% of your daily fiber needs (18).

Not only does fiber slow your digestive process to promote fullness, but it can also stabilize blood sugar to prevent hunger and cravings (19Trusted Source, 20Trusted Source).

Additionally, popcorn can help reduce appetite and enhance feelings of fullness more than many other popular snack foods.

In fact, one study in 35 people observed that those who ate 100 calories of popcorn were fuller and more satisfied than those who ate

150 calories of potato chips (21Trusted Source).

However, keep in mind that these benefits apply to air-popped popcorn. Many ready-made varieties are prepared with a lot of unhealthy fats, artificial flavorings and added salt or sugar, which greatly increases the calorie content.

SUMMARYPopcorn is high in fiber, which can slow your digestion and stabilize blood sugar. It also reduces hunger and promotes satisfaction better than other snacks.

7. Chia Seeds

Often hailed as a serious superfood, chia seeds pack a high amount of protein and fiber into a low number of calories.

A 1-ounce (28-gram) serving of chia seeds provides 137 calories, 4.4 grams of protein and a whopping 10.6 grams of fiber (22).

Chia seeds are especially high in soluble fiber, a type of fiber that absorbs liquid and swells in your stomach to promote feelings of fullness (23Trusted Source).

In fact, some research observes that chia seeds can absorb 10–12 times their weight in water, moving slowly through your digestive tract to keep you feeling full (24).

Adding a serving or two of chia seeds to your daily diet can curb cravings and reduce appetite.

In one study in 24 adults, those who consumed yogurt with added chia seeds reported decreased hunger, less desire for sugary foods and enhanced feelings of fullness compared to the control group (25Trusted Source).

SUMMARYChia seeds are loaded with soluble fiber, which can keep you feeling full throughout the day.

8. Fish

Fish is rich in protein and heart-healthy fats.

For instance, a 3-ounce (85-gram) serving of cod provides over 15 grams of protein and under 70 calories (26).

Some research points out that increasing protein intake can decrease appetite and reduce levels of ghrelin, the hormone that stimulates hunger (16Trusted Source, 27Trusted Source).

What's more, fish protein may be especially beneficial for reducing hunger levels and appetite.

One study evaluating the effects of beef, chicken and fish protein showed that fish protein had the greatest impact on feelings of fullness (28Trusted Source).

To cut calorie consumption even further, opt for lean fish like cod, flounder, halibut or sole over higher-calorie options like salmon, sardines or mackerel.

SUMMARYFish is high in protein, which can increase feelings of fullness and reduce appetite and hunger.

9. Cottage Cheese

Cottage cheese is a great source of protein and an excellent snack for those looking to lose weight.

One cup (226 grams) of low-fat cottage cheese packs about 28 grams of protein and just 163 calories (29).

Multiple studies demonstrate that upping your protein intake from foods like cottage cheese can decrease appetite and hunger levels (16Trusted Source, 27Trusted Source).

Some research also suggests that eating protein can slow the emptying of your stomach to prolong feelings of fullness (30Trusted Source, 31Trusted Source).

What's more, one study even found that cottage cheese and eggs had similar effects on fullness in 30 healthy adults (32Trusted Source).

SUMMARYCottage cheese is high in protein, which can decrease appetite and keep you feeling full.

10. Potatoes

Potatoes are often dismissed as unhealthy and harmful due to their association with high-fat french fries and potato chips.

However, the truth is that potatoes can be a filling and nutritious part of a healthy diet.

One medium baked potato with the skin contains 161 calories but provides 4 grams each of protein and fiber as well (33).

In fact, a study evaluating the effects of certain foods on satiety — or fullness — ranked boiled potatoes as the most filling, with a score of 323 on the satiety index — nearly seven times higher than croissants (34Trusted Source).

Animal and human studies indicate that the filling effects of potatoes may involve potato protease inhibitors, which are compounds that can reduce appetite and decrease food intake to boost fullness (35Trusted Source, 36Trusted Source).

SUMMARYPotatoes rank as one of the world's most filling foods and supply a specific compound that may decrease appetite and food intake.

11. Lean Meat

Lean meat can efficiently reduce hunger and appetite between meals.

Lean meats like chicken, turkey and low-fat cuts of red meat are low in calories but loaded with protein.

For example, 4 ounces (112 grams) of cooked chicken breast contains about 185 calories and 35 grams of protein.

Research suggests that insufficient protein intake could increase hunger and appetite while eating more protein can reduce calorie intake and hunger levels (37Trusted Source, 38Trusted Source, 39Trusted Source).

In one study, people who ate a high-protein meal including meat consumed 12% less food by weight at dinner than those who ate a high-carb, meatless meal (40Trusted Source).

SUMMARYLean meats are high in protein, which can reduce calorie intake and hunger.

12. Legumes

Because of their high protein and fiber content, legumes such as beans, peas and lentils can be incredibly filling.

One cup (198 grams) of cooked lentils provides about 230 calories, as well as 15.6 grams of fiber and nearly 18 grams of protein (41).

Multiple studies prove that legumes have a powerful effect on hunger and appetite.

One study in 43 young men noted that a high-protein meal with beans and peas increased feelings of fullness and reduced appetite and hunger more than a high-protein meal with veal and pork (42Trusted Source).

Another review of nine studies reported that people felt 31% more full after eating pulses, a type of legume, compared to high-carb meals of pasta and bread (43Trusted Source).

SUMMARYLegumes, which are high in protein and fiber, are associated with reduced appetite and hunger, as well as increased feelings of fullness.

13. Watermelon

Watermelon has a high water content to keep you hydrated and full while supplying a minimal number of calories.

One cup (152 grams) of diced watermelon contains 46 calories alongside an assortment of essential micronutrients like vitamins A and C (44).

Eating foods with a low calorie density, such as watermelon, has been shown to have similar effects on feelings of fullness and hunger compared to high-calorie-density foods (45Trusted Source, 46Trusted Source).

Plus, foods with a lower calorie density have been linked to lower body weight and decreased calorie intake (47Trusted Source).

In fact, in one study in 49 women, replacing oat cookies with an equal number of calories from fruit significantly reduced calorie intake and body weight (48Trusted Source).

SUMMARYWatermelon's high water content and low calorie density could promote fullness and reduce calorie intake.

The Bottom Line

Cutting back on calories doesn't mean you have to constantly feel hungry or unsatisfied between meals.

Eating a wide variety of filling foods with plenty of protein and fiber can fight cravings and decrease hunger to make weight loss easier than ever.

Paired with an active lifestyle and well-rounded diet, these low-calorie foods can keep you feeling satisfied throughout the day.

Calorie Density — How to Lose Weight Eating More Food

Calorie density describes the number of calories in a given volume or weight of food.

Understanding how it works can help you lose weight and improve your diet (1Trusted Source).

What's more, focusing on low-calorie-density foods allows you to eat a large volume of food while still cutting back on calories (2Trusted Source, 3Trusted Source, 4Trusted Source).

This can have many health benefits, including increased nutrient intake and weight loss.

This article explains everything you need to know about calorie density.

www.ingramcontent.com/pod-product-compliance
Lightning Source LLC
Chambersburg PA
CBHW061015260726
48661CB00005B/2201